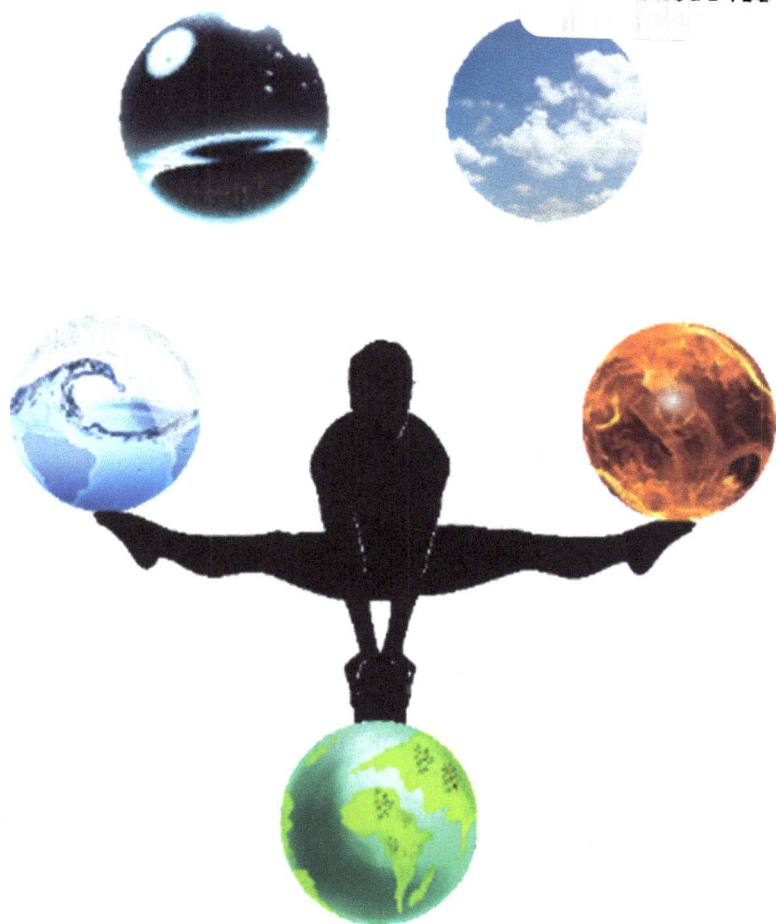

You Playbook

by Cynthia Schaefer
https://www.flurbanparadise.com

Find me on Amazon:
https://amzn.to/434aRxp

This book is dedicated to all of us who have struggled with finding a way to be healthy and whole.

Publisher: Flurban Paradise
4786 SW 72nd Ave.
Davie, Florida 33314
https://www.flurbanparadise.com

Special thanks to my content editor, and to all who have inspired me along the way.
Liliane V Abello [https://linkedin.com/in/lily-abello]

ISBN: 9798989391615

Table of Contents

Medical Disclaimer

This book is intended for informational purposes only and does not serve as a replacement for professional medical advice, diagnosis, or treatment.

The author and publisher are not medical professionals; the information presented herein is based on traditional knowledge, personal experiences, and research.

Always consult with a qualified healthcare provider or herbalist before changing your diet, medications, or health routines, especially when introducing new herbs or supplements. Some herbs can interact with medications or have side effects.

Every individual's body is unique, and what works for one person may not work for another. Never disregard professional medical advice or delay seeking it because of something you have read in this book.

If you think you may have a medical emergency, call your doctor, go to the emergency department, or call emergency services immediately.

The author and publisher disclaim any liability or loss, personal or otherwise, resulting from the procedures and information presented in this book.

Welcome to your You Playbook!

The purpose of this journal is to allow you to track your progress and record the amazing journey you are about to embark upon.

This is week one of your journey.

By the end of the first week, you will understand what elements are primary in your base constitution and what elements might be out of balance. The first series of questions is about your base constitution.

You want to answer these questions based on what is usual for you. For example, if you've been cold most of your life but recently feel warmer, answer based on what is usual, not what might have changed recently.

You'll total up the numbers of your answers for each element. You might want to take this test multiple times as you begin implementing your Secret Formula; you may find changes. Sometimes, our primary element isn't revealed immediately if we've been out of balance for a long time.

There will be a different test for imbalances. We will look at those later.

WEEK 1: Who are you?

Air Element:

1. How often do you find your mind jumping from one thought to another?

(1) Rarely
(2) Occasionally
(3) Sometimes
(4) Often
(5) Always

2. How would you describe your physical activity level?

(1) Sedentary
(2) Light
(3) Moderate
(4) Active
(5) Very Active

3. How quickly do you tend to speak?

(1) Very slowly
(2) Slowly
(3) At a moderate pace
(4) Quickly
(5) Very quickly

4. How would you describe your body frame?

(1) Large/Heave
(2) Somewhat large
(3) Medium
(4) Slim
(5) Very slim

5. How quickly do you adapt to new situations?

(1) Very slowly
(2) Slowly
(3) At a moderate pace
(4) Quickly
(5) Very quickly

6. How often do you experience anxiety or nervousness?

(1) Rarely
(2) Occasionally
(3) Sometimes
(4) Often
(5) Always

7. How would you describe your sleeping pattern?

(1) Deep sleeper
(2) Somewhat deep sleeper
(3) Average sleeper
(4) Light sleeper
(5) Very light sleeper

Earth Element:

1. How strong is your attachment to material possessions?

(1) Very low
(2) Low
(3) Moderate
(4) High
(5) Very high

2. How would you describe your digestive system?

(1) Very weak
(2) Weak
(3) Average
(4) Strong
(5) Very strong

3. How stable do you consider your emotions to be?

(1) Very unstable
(2) Unstable
(3) Neutral
(4) Stable
(5) Very stable

4. How would you describe your pace in daily activities?

(1) Very fast
(2) Fast
(3) Moderate
(4) Slow
(5) Very slow

5. How connected do you feel to nature and the environment?

(1) Not at all
(2) Slightly
(3) Moderately
(4) Quite a bit
(5) Extremely

6. How easy is it for you to gain weight?

(1) Very hard
(2) Hard
(3) Neutral
(4) Easy
(5) Very easy

7. How would you describe your skin type?

(1) Very dry
(2) Dry
(3) Normal
(4) Oily
(5) Very oily

Ether Element:

1. How imaginative or creative would you say you are?

(1) Not at all
(2) A little
(3) Somewhat
(4) Quite
(5) Extremely

2. How frequently do you meditate or engage in deep reflection?

(1) Never
(2) Rarely
(3) Sometimes
(4) Often
(5) Daily

3. How would you describe your connection to spirituality or the metaphysical?

(1) Non-existent
(2) Slight
(3) Moderate
(4) Strong
(5) Very strong

4. How often do you experience feelings of detachment or space-iness?

(1) Never
(2) Rarely
(3) Sometimes
(4) Often
(5) Always

5. How easy is it for you to forgive others?

(1) Very difficult
(2) Difficult
(3) Neutral
(4) Easy
(5) Very easy

6. How receptive are you to new ideas and perspectives?

(1) Not at all
(2) Slightly
(3) Moderately
(4) Quite
(5) Extremely

7. How often do you find yourself daydreaming?

(1) Never
(2) Rarely
(3) Sometimes
(4) Often
(5) Always

Water Element:

1. How would you describe your emotional sensitivity?

(1) Very low
(2) Low
(3) Moderate
(4) High
(5) Very high

2. How good are you at going with the flow in unexpected situations?

(1) Very poor
(2) Poor
(3) Average
(4) Good
(5) Excellent

3. How would you describe your fluid intake daily?

(1) Very insufficient
(2) Insufficient
(3) Adequate
(4) More than enough
(5) Excessive

4. How connected do you feel to your emotions and intuition?

(1) Not at all
(2) Slightly
(3) Moderately
(4) Quite a bit
(5) Extremely

5. How would you describe your ability to relate to others emotionally?

(1) Very poor
(2) Poor
(3) Average
(4) Good
(5) Excellent

6. How often do you cry or feel moved to tears?

(1) Never
(2) Rarely
(3) Sometimes
(4) Often
(5) Very frequently

7. How would you describe your dreams?

(1) Non-existent
(2) Sparse and plain
(3) Moderate
(4) Vivid
(5) Waking dreams

Fire Element:

1. How would you describe your metabolic rate?

(1) Very slow
(2) Slow
(3) Moderate
(4) Fast
(5) Very fast

2. How often do you find yourself taking initiative and leadership in group settings?

(1) Never
(2) Rarely
(3) Sometimes
(4) Often
(5) Always

3. How would you describe your approach to completing tasks and goals?

(1) Laid-back
(2) Somewhat relaxed
(3) Moderate
(4) Proactive
(5) Very proactive

4. How would you describe your digestive system?

(1) Weak
(2) Somewhat weak
(3) Moderate
(4) Strong
(5) Very strong

5. How often do you find yourself feeling warm or preferring cooler environments?

(1) Never
(2) Rarely
(3) Sometimes
(4) Often
(5) Always

6. How would you rate your passion and enthusiasm in your daily activities?

(1) Very low
(2) Low
(3) Moderate
(4) High
(5) Very high

7. How often do you find yourself taking risks or seeking new adventures?

(1) Never
(2) Rarely
(3) Sometimes
(4) Often
(5) Always

This page is for you to add up your totals and make notes.

Totals:

Air_____

Earth_____

Ether_____

Water_____

Fire_____

Conclusion: My primary element(s) are:

_____

_____

Take this information and put it in the I AM section that begins on page 49.

Now, Read about your primary element(s) below. Take your time and reflect on what feels true to you. Then, go to the I AM section on page 49 and fill in the playbook.

Air Element

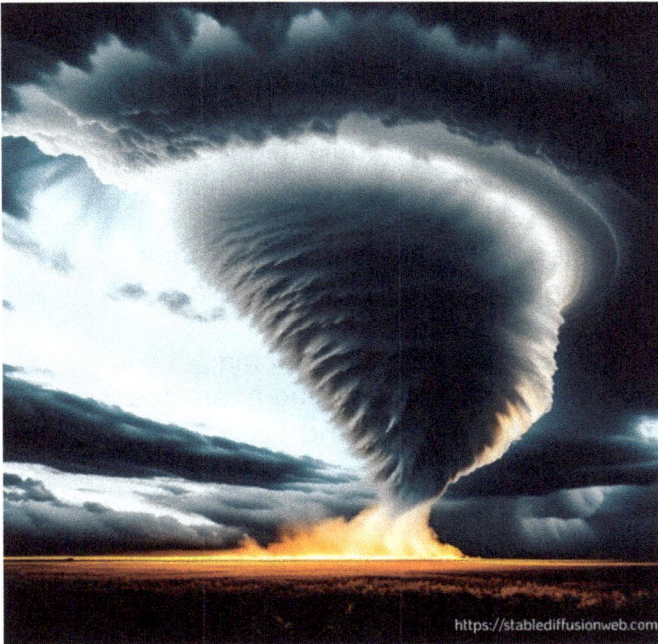

https://stablediffusionweb.com

1. General Overview:

Air represents movement, change, and lightness. It embodies the qualities of flexibility, communication, and intellect. It's associated with thoughts, ideas, and the breath.

2. Strengths and Benefits:

Adaptability: Those with a strong air element can easily adjust to different situations and changes.
Communication: Air enhances the ability to express oneself and to connect with others.
Creativity and Ideas: A heightened

sense of imagination and a rich realm of ideas often dominate the mind.

3. Challenges and Growth Opportunities:

Grounding: Air individuals might struggle to feel grounded or focused, often "in their heads."

Consistency: Maintaining consistency can be challenging due to its changeable nature.

Growth Opportunity: Developing mindfulness practices or grounding exercises can help anchor their energy and cultivate stability.

Earth Element

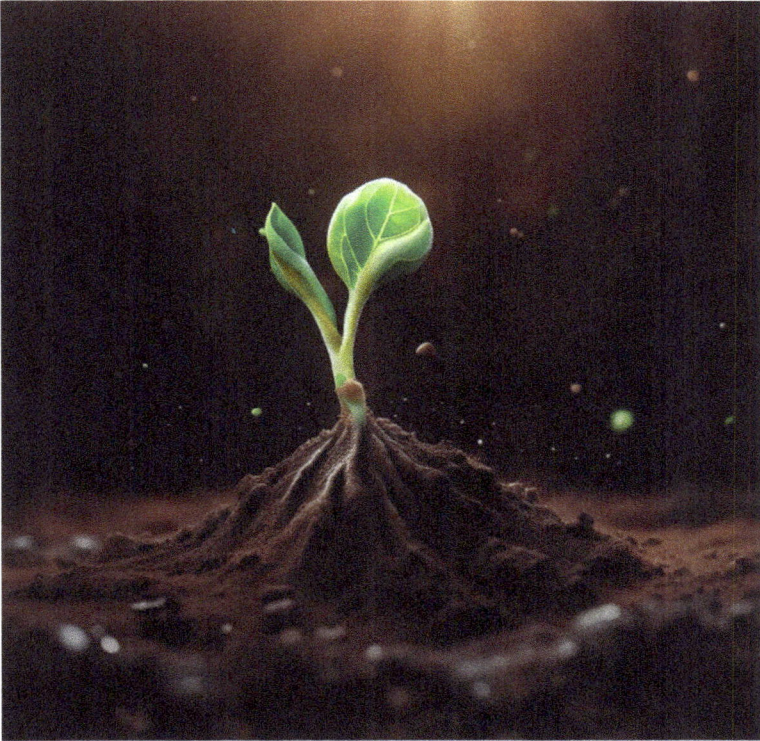

1. General Overview:

Earth represents stability, grounded-ness, and nourishment. It's associated with the physical body, nature, and the sense of touch.

2. Strengths and Benefits:

Stability: Those dominated by the Earth element tend to be reliable and consistent.
Practicality: They possess a grounded approach to life and make decisions based on

realism.

Nurturing: Earth individuals often have a strong nurturing instinct, providing care and stability to those around them.

3. Challenges and Growth Opportunities:

Resistance to Change: They may struggle with change or anything that disrupts their stability.

Tendency to be Overly Cautious: Might miss opportunities due to overemphasizing safety or security.

Growth Opportunity: Embracing change and cultivating flexibility can bring a renewed sense of freedom and growth.

Ether Element

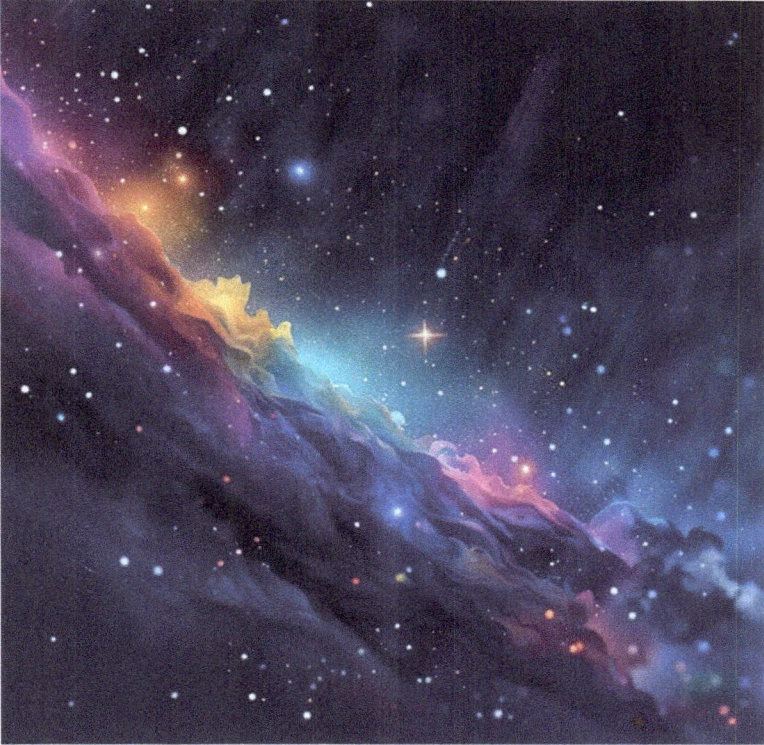

1. General Overview:

Ether, also called "Space," represents the vastness, the emptiness, and the spiritual realm. It's the bridge between the physical and the non-physical.

2. Strengths and Benefits:

Intuition and Insight: Ether-dominated individuals often possess deep intuition and spiritual insights.

Open-mindedness: They are typically open to new ideas and are receptive listeners.

Connection to the Spiritual: Often have a heightened sense of spirituality or connection to higher realms.

3. Challenges and Growth Opportunities:

Grounding: May struggle to stay connected with the tangible, getting lost in thought or daydreams.

Detachment: Might feel distant or detached from the world around them.

Growth Opportunity: Engaging with the physical realm, like through tactile activities, can enhance their connection to the world.

Water Element

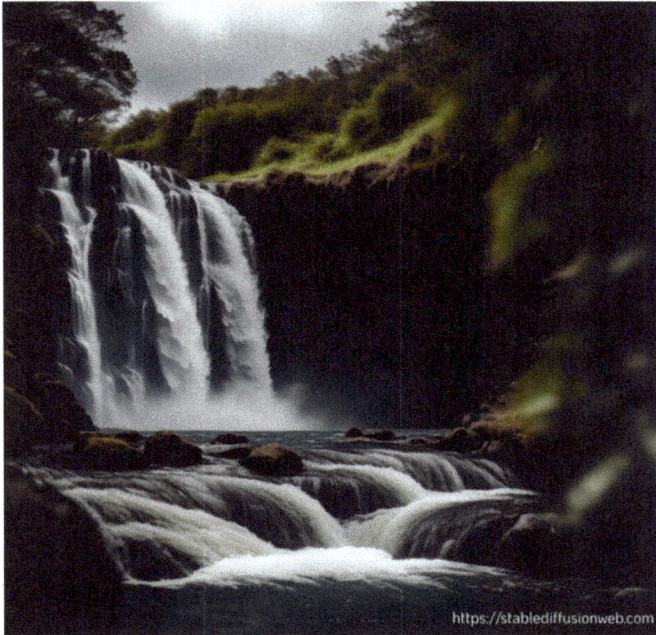

1. General Overview:

Water represents fluidity, emotions, and intuition. It's associated with the heart, feelings, and the ability to connect emotionally.

2. Strengths and Benefits:

     Empathy: Water individuals are often deeply empathic and understanding.

     Emotional Depth: They can navigate the depths of emotions, both theirs and others.

     Receptivity: They are typically open and receptive, allowing them to connect deeply with others.

3. Challenges and Growth Opportunities:

Overwhelm: Can easily become overwhelmed by their own or others emotions.

Boundary Issues: Might struggle to set boundaries, absorbing others' feelings.

Growth Opportunity: Learning emotional regulation and setting clear boundaries can ensure they don't deplete their energy.

Fire Element

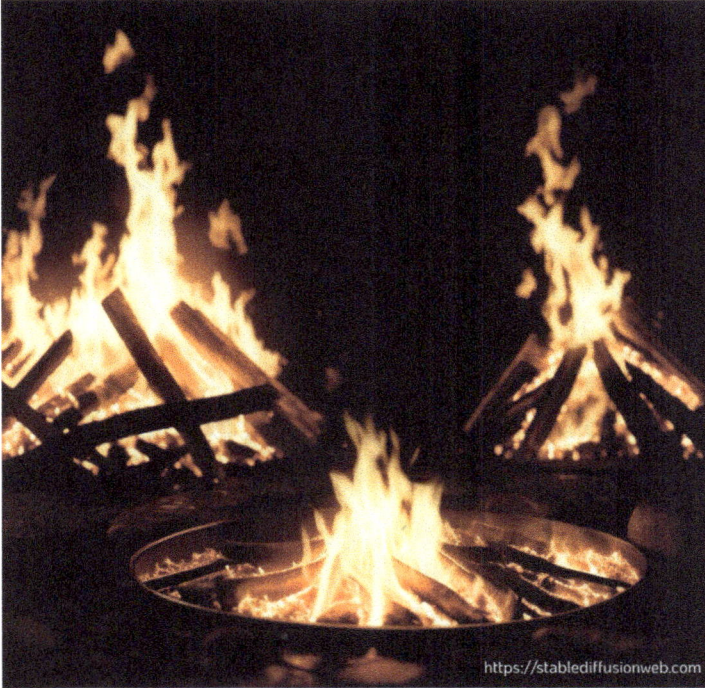

https://stablediffusionweb.com

1. General Overview:

Fire represents transformation, passion, and dynamism. It's associated with energy, drive, and the will.

2. Strengths and Benefits:

Passion: Those with a strong fire element are often deeply passionate and enthusiastic.
Transformation: They possess the power to transform and renew situations.
Leadership: Naturally assertive, they often

take leadership roles and inspire others.

3. Challenges and Growth Opportunities:

Impulsivity: Might act without thinking or let their passions override reason.
Burnout: Their intense energy can lead to burnout if not channeled properly.
Growth Opportunity: Cultivating patience and reflection can help harness their energy in a balanced way.

Now, take some time and reflect on this. The element(s) with the highest numbers will be primary for you. It is not unusual for a person to have two equally primary elements. Go to page 49 and fill in the first part of the I AM section.

Be sure not to get caught up in describing an element as good or bad. Like everything in life, every element has two sides to the coin. We are learning about the properties and using them to adjust ourselves to be the most balanced and highest expression of ourselves.

When trying to understand an element, it is good to think about how it is expressed in nature. Water is important for all of life, but too much water in the wrong place can be catastrophic.

A campfire and a forest fire are very different things. A warm summer breeze is nothing like a tornado. You get the picture. Keeping the elements within us in balance helps keep our body in homeostasis.

Homeostasis is just a fancy word for balance. Every element is both good and bad.

WEEK 2: Imbalances

Imbalances can be too much or too little, but we will work from the standpoint of having an imbalanced element that is too much in this format. Correcting too much fire, for example, will also correct too little earth and/or water.

Now, let's look for any imbalances. You'll do the same thing with these questions, but now we are looking to understand things happening now but haven't been part of the way you usually are.

Air Element:

1. How often do you experience dry skin or dry eyes?

(1) Never
(2) Rarely
(3) Sometimes
(4) Often
(5) Always

2. How frequently do you find yourself lost in thoughts, unable to focus on the present moment?

(1) Never
(2) Rarely
(3) Sometimes
(4) Often
(5) Always

3. How often do you struggle with insomnia or restless sleep?

(1) Never
(2) Rarely
(3) Sometimes
(4) Often
(5) Always

4. How prone are you to experiencing anxiety and nervousness?

(1) Never
(2) Rarely
(3) Sometimes
(4) Often
(5) Always

5. How often do you have digestive issues like bloating or gas?

(1) Never
(2) Rarely
(3) Sometimes
(4) Often
(5) Always

Earth Element:

1. How often do you feel overly attached or possessive towards things or people?

(1) Never
(2) Rarely
(3) Sometimes
(4) Often
(5) Always

2. How frequently do you experience sluggish digestion or constipation?

(1) Never
(2) Rarely
(3) Sometimes
(4) Often
(5) Always

3. How often do you feel stuck, unable to embrace change or new experiences?

(1) Never
(2) Rarely
(3) Sometimes
(4) Often
(5) Always

4. How often do you experience feelings of lethargy or lack of motivation?

(1) Never
(2) Rarely
(3) Sometimes
(4) Often
(5) Always

5. How frequently do you find yourself overeating or craving salty and sweet foods?

(1) Never
(2) Rarely
(3) Sometimes
(4) Often
(5) Always

Ether Element:

1. How often do you feel disconnected or spaced out, losing touch with reality?

(1) Never
(2) Rarely
(3) Sometimes
(4) Often
(5) Always

2. How often do you experience difficulties in communicating your thoughts clearly to others?

(1) Never
(2) Rarely
(3) Sometimes
(4) Often
(5) Always

3. How frequently do you struggle with feeling grounded and stable in your daily life?

(1) Never
(2) Rarely
(3) Sometimes
(4) Often
(5) Always

4. How often do you feel uninterested or apathetic towards physical activities or the material world?

(1) Never
(2) Rarely
(3) Sometimes
(4) Often
(5) Always

5. How frequently do you experience feelings of loneliness or isolation?
(1) Never
(2) Rarely
(3) Sometimes
(4) Often
(5) Always

Water Element:

1. How often do you feel emotionally overwhelmed, as if you carry too much emotional weight?

(1) Never
(2) Rarely
(3) Sometimes
(4) Often
(5) Always

2. How frequently do you experience fluid-related issues such as water retention or urinary problems?

(1) Never
(2) Rarely
(3) Sometimes
(4) Often
(5) Always

3. How often do you find it difficult to set boundaries and say no when necessary?

(1) Never
(2) Rarely
(3) Sometimes
(4) Often
(5) Always

4. How frequently do you experience cold hands and feet, or a general feeling of being cold?

(1) Never
(2) Rarely
(3) Sometimes
(4) Often
(5) Always

5. How often do you struggle with feelings of insecurity or fear?

(1) Never
(2) Rarely
(3) Sometimes
(4) Often
(5) Always

Fire Element:

1. How frequently do you experience inflammatory issues such as redness, heat, or swelling in the body?

(1) Never
(2) Rarely
(3) Sometimes
(4) Often
(5) Always

2. How often do you find yourself experiencing bouts of anger or irritability?

(1) Never
(2) Rarely
(3) Sometimes
(4) Often
(5) Always

3. How frequently do you struggle with impulsive behavior or making rash decisions?

(1) Never
(2) Rarely
(3) Sometimes
(4) Often
(5) Always

4. How often do you experience heartburn, acid reflux, or other fiery digestive issues?

(1) Never
(2) Rarely
(3) Sometimes
(4) Often
(5) Always

5. How often do you struggle with feelings of jealousy or envy?

(1) Never
(2) Rarely
(3) Sometimes
(4) Often
(5) Always

We'll use the same scoring system:

Totals:

Air_____

Earth_____

Ether_____

Water_____

Fire_____

The higher numbers will point to your imbalances. When we begin our vibrant wellness journey, it is common to have many or all of the elements out of balance. You want to work with the highest scores first.

Put those results in your I AM section in your You Playbook and complete the section under WEEK 2 that begins on page 30.

If your primary element is also one of your imbalanced ones, and there is no clear leader in your other elemental imbalances, work with your primary first.

Many times, you can work on two imbalances at once. Too much fire and too little water can be the same imbalance. Add water, and the fire gets reduced.

Earth imbalances almost always affect digestion.

Root vegetables are full of prebiotics and fiber. If constipation is a problem; prioritize that, as poor gut health can cause many other problems. How do I balance all this?

Now, we get to the heart of the matter. Some of this will be intuitive. Remember, nobody knows your body like you do.

Walking the Tightrope

You'll find breathwork, movement, and intake recommendations for each imbalance below. You can mix and match and try different combinations. Correcting an imbalance doesn't happen overnight. Take your time with this, and find your center.

My YouTube channel has videos of each of these, so please subscribe. You can find me here: https://bit.ly/Flurban. There will be general content on achieving vibrant wellness on the channel as well as specific videos for the movements and breathwork recommended here.

Air Element

Breathwork:
Alternate Nostril Breathing (Nadi Shodhana): Helps balance the brain's left and right hemispheres and create a sense of calm.

Bhramari Breath (Bee Breath): This can be soothing and helps to reduce anxiety, a common issue with air imbalance.

Movement:
Yoga poses promote grounding, such as Mountain Pose and Child's Pose.

Slow, controlled Tai Chi movements can help in grounding the air element.

Food:
Root vegetables, like carrots, beets, and sweet potatoes, can promote grounding.

Warm and cooked foods: Avoid raw and cold foods to counteract excess air element.

Affirmations:
"I am grounded, focused, and at peace with the world around me."

"With each breath, I draw in stability and release uncertainty."

Earth Element

Breathwork:
Kapalabhati (Skull Shining Breath): Helps energize the body and counter lethargy.

Sitali Breath (Cooling Breath): This can help bring a light and fresh perspective, mitigating the stagnant energy of excess earth.

Movement:
Backbends in yoga, like Cobra Pose or Upward Facing Dog, can introduce energy and fluidity.

Dynamic dancing: Encourage fluid movement and break up stagnation.

Food:
Leafy greens, like kale and spinach, can counter heaviness.

Spicy foods: These can help in stimulating digestion and breaking up stagnation.

Affirmations:
"I am adaptable, flowing effortlessly through changes and challenges."

"I nurture myself with loving kindness, welcoming lightness and vitality into my body."

Ether Element

Breathwork:
Ujjayi Breath (Ocean Breath): This can help ground and focus the mind.

Dirga Breath (Three-Part Breath): Helps connect with the physical body and ground excess ether.

Movement:
Stability and balancing poses, like Tree Pose or Warrior III in yoga, can help in grounding excess ether elements.

Strength training: Focus on exercises that build muscle and connect with the physical body.

Food:
Protein-rich foods, like legumes and lean meats, can help in grounding.

Root vegetables: Incorporate more grounding foods to balance excess ether.

Affirmations:
"I am connected to my physical presence and honor the space I occupy."

"I am grounded in the here and now, embracing the tangible and the real with open arms."

Water Element

Breathwork:
Bhastrika (Bellows Breath): This can be energizing and helps in reducing excess water.

Surya Bhedana (Right Nostril Breathing): Activates the fiery energy, balancing excess water.

Movement:
Twisting yoga poses, like Spinal Twist, help in reducing water retention.

Cardiovascular exercises include jogging or cycling to stimulate heat and reduce excess water.

Food:
Diuretic foods like asparagus and celery can help in reducing water retention.

Bitter foods: such as kale and dandelion greens can help in balancing excess water.

Affirmations:
"I am fluid, releasing what no longer serves me with grace and ease."

"I foster inner warmth and fire, balancing fluidity with purposeful action."

Fire Element

Breathwork:
Sheetali Breath (Cooling Breath): Helps in cooling down excess fire.

Chandra Bhedana (Left Nostril Breathing): Activates the cooling energy, balancing excess fire.

Movement:
Yin yoga: Slow, restorative postures can help in cooling the system.

Swimming: A cooling and gentle exercise to reduce fire.

Food:
Cooling foods: such as cucumbers, melons, and leafy greens can help reduce fire imbalance.

Mint or chamomile tea: Can have a cooling effect on the body.

Affirmations:
"I am calm, cool, and collected, harnessing the fiery energy within me with wisdom and restraint."

"I radiate a peaceful glow, offering warmth and light to myself and others."

Know Yourself

Everything has positives and negatives. Learning your strengths and weaknesses allows you to grow mindfully.

We lean into our strengths and try to cover up our weaknesses. There is a saying that a chain is only as strong as its weakest link. We are best served by strengthening our weaknesses. This gives us balance.

I wrote this book to give us all a different way of looking at ourselves and the people around us. We could all use more true self-love and acceptance, more understanding of how to stay healthy and balanced in a world that seems to be spinning faster and faster.

If you were standing before me, I would tell you to love yourself. I would remind you that you came here with gifts, talents, and a purpose. I would ask you to treat yourself with as much care, nurturing, and patience as you treat your most beloved.

Vibrant health is possible at any age. No matter how far down the road of chronic illness, you can improve by choosing differently. You can feel better and have more energy and love of life.

As you take this journey, there will be times when the changes are challenging. Remember Future You, and know you have what it takes to make Future You come true. One day, you will wake up and realize that Future You is here, and it only gets better.

I AM

Who am I?

My primary element is: _____

The positive ways that this element works for me in my body are:

_____

_____

_____

_____

_____

The positive ways this element works for me in my thoughts and emotions are:

_____

_____

_____

_____

_____

The challenges this element presents for me in
my body are:

_____

_____

_____

_____

_____

The challenges this element presents for me in
my thoughts and emotions are:

_____

_____

_____

_____

_____

The growth opportunities this presents for me to overcome the challenges are:

_____

_____

_____

_____

_____

When I overcome the challenges, I will be (Examples might be calmer, more decisive, stronger physically, etc.)

_____

_____

_____

_____

_____

On the following few pages, try some artwork.

Doodle, use colored pencils, pen, or paint, and let yourself free flow. Let your subconscious speak to you about this element and how it speaks to you and your understanding of yourself.

You can also use the following few pages to jot down thoughts and impressions.

If you have equal elements, do the exercises again with your second element. If you don't, skip this part. Or you can use it for your secondary element.

My primary (secondary) element is:

_____

The positive way that this element works for me in
my body are:

_____

_____

_____

_____

The positive way this element works for me in my
thoughts and emotions are:

_____

_____

_____

_____

_____

The challenges this element presents for me in my body are:

_____

_____

_____

_____

_____

The challenges this element presents for me in my thoughts and emotions are:

_____

_____

_____

_____

_____

The growth opportunities this presents for me to overcome the challenges are:

_____

_____

_____

_____

_____

When I overcome the challenges, I will be (Examples might be calmer, more decisive, stronger physically, etc.)

_____

_____

_____

_____

_____

_____

How I feel about my primary element(s):

_____

_____

_____

_____

Reflections about my primary element(s):
(How did it shape you? How will your life change
because you know your elemental strengths and
weaknesses?) How do you feel about it?)

_____

_____

_____

_____

_____

_____

_____

_____

_____

Artwork and impressions of my primary element
(or secondary):

WEEK 3: Finding my balance

My primary imbalance(s) are:

_____

_____

_____

_____

_____

The ways that this imbalance has been made stronger by my actions are (e.g., Feeding fire with too much stimulation, encouraging water by watching movies that you know will make you cry, etc.):

_____

_____

_____

_____

_____

The impact of this imbalance on my body and mind has been (can't sleep, overly emotional, constipated, etc.)

_____

_____

_____

_____

_____

Thinking intuitively, the things I can do to correct my imbalances are:

_____

_____

_____

_____

_____

I can be more aware of how this element might tend towards imbalance in the future by:

_____

_____

_____

_____

_____

Artwork or words that express my thoughts and feelings related to this imbalance:

WEEK 4: Making it Real

The things that surprised me about my primary element(s) and imbalance(s) were:

_____

_____

_____

_____

_____

A permanent change I will make:

_____

_____

_____

_____

_____

This next section is meant to be a shortcut and a way for you to anchor your knowledge of the techniques that work for you. You can answer for some or all of the elements. This will help you to connect the imbalance to the balancing technique.

The breathing techniques I will practice:

When I am out of balance in my fire element are:

_____

_____

_____

_____

When I am out of balance in my air element are:

_____

_____

_____

_____

When I am out of balance in my water element are:

_____

_____

_____

_____

_____

When I am out of balance in my ether element are:

_____

_____

_____

_____

When I am out of balance in my earth element are:

_____

_____

_____

_____

The movements I will practice:

When I am out of balance in my fire element are:

_____

_____

_____

_____

When I am out of balance in my air element are:

_____

_____

_____

_____

When I am out of balance in my water element are:

_____

_____

_____

_____

When I am out of balance in my ether element are:

_____

_____

_____

_____

When I am out of balance in my earth element are:

_____

_____

_____

_____

The foods, spices, and herbs I will choose:

When I am out of balance in my fire element are:

_____

_____

_____

_____

When I am out of balance in my air element are:

_____

_____

_____

_____

When I am out of balance in my water element are:

_____

_____

_____

_____

When I am out of balance in my ether element are:

_____

_____

_____

_____

When I am out of balance in my earth element are:

_____

_____

_____

_____

The thoughts/affirmations that are good for me:

When I am out of balance in my fire element are:

_____

_____

_____

_____

When I am out of balance in my air element are:

_____

_____

_____

_____

When I am out of balance in my water element are:

_____

_____

_____

_____

When I am out of balance in my ether element are:

_____

_____

_____

_____

When I am out of balance in my earth element are:

_____

_____

_____

_____

The changes I have made so far:

_____

_____

_____

_____

_____

The changes I have noticed so far:

_____

_____

_____

_____

_____

WEEK 5: Assess, Reflect, Adjust

This week is all about you tracking your progress, assessing what's working and what's not, and making the adjustments to go forward. By now, your initial changes will have become routine and easy, and it's time for a deeper look.

The things that I changed that were easy were:

_____

_____

_____

_____

_____

The things that I changed that were hard were:

_____

_____

_____

_____

_____

The things that I still want to change are:

_____

_____

_____

_____

In order of importance, these are the things I will work on this week:

_____

_____

_____

_____

Write a promise to yourself about the changes you are making this week. If you don't have any changes you are ready to make, then write a love letter to yourself about how far you've already come:

_____

_____

_____

_____

Use this space to create artwork or writings that speak about where you are on your journey and where you are going:

WEEK 6: Take it to the Street

Find a friend! By now, the people around you have noticed the changes in you. This is a good time to share what you are doing. Offer to loan them the book or help them take the assessment tests. Many times, we have friends and family who have similar imbalances.

One of the best parts of a journey to vibrant health is the chance to reach out to someone else. When you walk the talk, people listen more closely to your words. Be an ambassador of vibrant health. We all gain when someone becomes stronger, happier, and healthier.

I think my friend(s) _____

_____

might benefit from taking this journey for themselves.

I think my family member(s) _____

_____

might benefit from taking this journey for themselves.

A new food(s) that I'm eating that I would like
to share with friends and family is:

_____

_____

_____

A breathing technique that I love and think
would help others is:

_____

_____

_____

_____

An activity that I love to do and would like
someone to do it with me is:

_____

_____

_____

_____

A group activity or team sport I'd like to try:

_____

_____

_____

_____

_____

Resources I can use to find these group
activities or team sports:

_____

_____

_____

_____

Class(es) I'd like to take to learn more about
food, spices or herbs is:

_____

_____

_____

_____

A movement class that I'd love to take is:

_____

_____

_____

_____

Read over your answers and make a list of the people you'd like to do things with and the classes, sports, or activities you'd like to do. Find out where you can take the classes or join the teams and DO it!

WEEK 7: Checking In

Take a moment and congratulate yourself! You've committed to vibrant wellness and are now a strong, empowered, and healthy human!

This is a good time to retake all the assessments. Before you do that, take an internal assessment. You might already know if you need to make some adjustments in some areas.

An area in which I may still have a minor imbalance is:

_____

_____

_____

_____

Some things I feel intuitively I could do to correct the minor imbalance above:

_____

_____

_____

_____

Retaking the assessments told me I was:

_____

_____

_____

_____

_____

I'm going to continue to work on:

_____

_____

_____

_____

_____

_____

It's all about you. Use the rest of the space to talk to Future You, or Prior You.

Journal feelings, things that worked or didn't work, or anything you'd like.

_____

_____

_____

_____

_____

_____

_____

_____

_____

_____

_____

_____

_____

_____

Congratulations on your courage in taking this journey!

www.ingramcontent.com/pod-product-compliance
Lightning Source LLC
Chambersburg PA
CBHW070027030426
42335CB00017B/2326